I0428413

Gluten-Free Club: Gluten-Free Secrets For Weight Loss

Gluten-Free Secrets to Weight Loss That You Wish You Knew

By Shari Darling

www.understandpublishing.com

For additional information please contact:

Understand Publishing (www.understandpublishing.com) at shariLdarling@gmail.com

Special Thanks to my Editor,

Deanna Shanti, Shanti Publishing

About Shari Darling

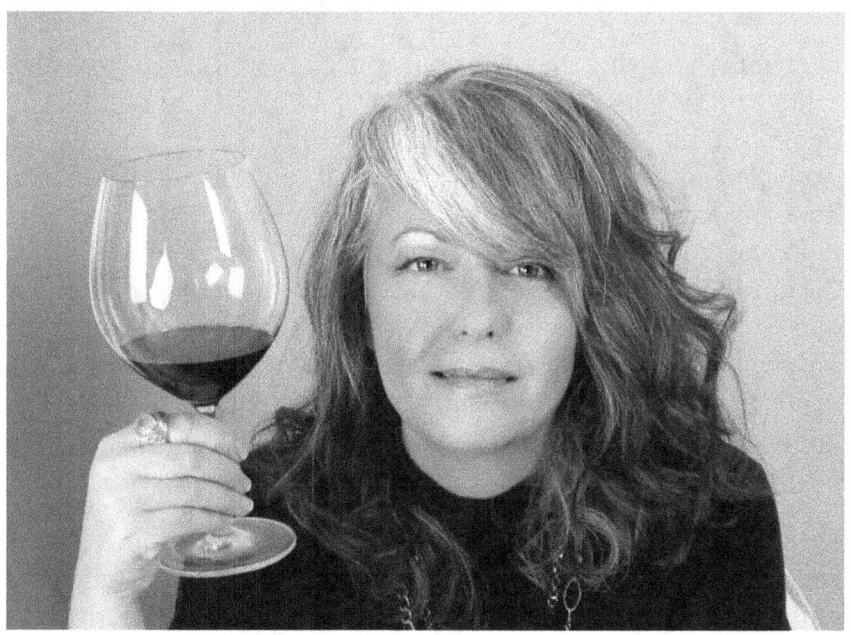

Hi, my name is Shari Darling.

I am a food and wine cookbook author, newspaper columnist, wine judge, restaurant reviewer and educator of wine and food. My website is www.understandpublishing.com

Quite by accident I discovered a few years ago that I am gluten-sensitive. At first I thought this discovery would hamper my work in wine and food. This is not the case at all.

The Gluten-Free lifestyle or 'diet' (which is not really the right word because I don't believe in dieting) will not require you to cut portions or count calories. It is not about starving your body of fats or carbohydrates. It is also not about weighing your food or removing bananas. It's mostly about eating a generally healthy diet of whole foods and finding substitutions to enjoy the foods you've always loved. Eat bread, just choose a Gluten-Free version and eat in moderation. Enjoy pasta? Then eat pasta, but find a decent Gluten-Free version and eat in moderation. The only strict rule is to avoid boxed and pre-prepared Gluten-

Free foods. There are also secrets to ensuring that the Gluten-Free diet will support you in losing weight.

I am not advocating that everyone must be on a Gluten-Free diet. I don't think wheat is bad. However, having read a plethora of books on the subject of wheat and Gluten-Free and having experienced the benefits of Gluten-Free first hand, I can honestly say it's the best choice for me and for anyone else who is experiencing side effects from gluten. I can tell you that a Gluten-Free diet has greatly contributed to both my husband and I shedding unwanted pounds. Although this was not the only contributor. We eat a healthy diet, watch food portions, drink alcohol moderately and exercise regularly as well. But going Gluten-Free really is super simple.

I discovered my gluten sensitivity after an evening of entertaining Gluten-Free friends. When entertaining I like to cater to my friends' specific culinary diets and requirements. I enjoy the challenge of meeting their dietary needs and surprising them with specialized, multi course meals paired with complementary wines.

About 4 years ago I decided to have a girlfriend and her husband over for a multi-course meal. My girlfriend is gluten- intolerant. So for the main entree I made homemade Gluten-Free lasagna accompanied by Gluten-Free garlic bread.

I had prepared enough lasagna for 12 people, hoping to wrap up the leftovers to give to my girlfriend to take home with her. We all enjoyed the lasagna so much we emptied the over-sized baking dish. When over-indulging on pasta and bread, I expect to wake up the next morning feeling hung-over, face and stomach bloated. I normally arise at 6 a.m. But after an evening of pasta I expect to wake up much later, closer to 8 am. It has always been this way. I have tolerated the effects of pasta and bread on my digestive system, believing the side effects came from the fact that pasta and bread are carbohydrates that makes everyone groggy.

The morning after this particular lasagna indulgence I woke up at 6:30 am and felt surprisingly alert. My stomach felt and looked flat and empty and was at peace. No grumbling. My face was normal, not bloated. This was the beginning of my awakening to the fact that I may have been gluten-sensitive.

I started eating Gluten-Free foods sporadically, not wanting to give up my love of pasta made with semolina flour and my addiction to all kinds of bread. But over time and with supermarkets implementing a whole section of Gluten-Free products, I started to eat Gluten-Free more often, then in time moved to a full lifestyle change. I walk 3 times a week for 3 miles and garden, as well. The regular routine of living Gluten-Free, eating smaller portions of the foods I love (just Gluten-Free versions), plus moderate exercise has motivated my 60 lb. weight loss.

I still indulge in pizza, burgers and spaghetti and meatballs. I just make sure I choose Gluten-Free dough.

I share my discoveries in the Gluten-Free Club on Facebook:

http://theglutenfreeclub.net/facebook

I advocate that a Gluten-Free diet can benefit everyone who is interested in healing the body and brain.

I've developed this book to give you access to the possibility of shedding those unwanted pounds by removing wheat and other gluten products from your lifestyle.

I am not a doctor. I am a Gluten-Free consumer. This e-book simply provides some simple and best practices, advice, tips and food suggestions I've obtained through my own gluten-sensitivity journey. Take what ideas work for you and be sure to consult your doctor.

To support you in your journey and to check out our other books in this genre and others go to www.understandpublishing.com and Click the icon called "Our Books"

Table of Contents

Introduction

I want to thank you and congratulate you for downloading the book, *Gluten-Free Secrets for Weight Loss*.

I wrote a book called Gluten-Free Made Simple. The information in this book is also contained here, in Gluten-Free Secrets for Weight Loss. So, don't waste your money by purchasing Gluten-Free Made Simple. There's no need.

This specific book contains the secrets – the information, tips, steps and strategies on how to successfully live a Gluten-Free lifestyle (or diet), potentially heal your body from ailments and provide you with the inspiration and most of all, lose weight!

In choosing to open this book, you've taken the first step to creating the possibility of a healthier and slimmer you! Remember, it's not the information in this guide that will make you lose weight. It is what you utilize from this guide that will make the difference. Only YOU can do the work.

Gluten-Free secrets for weight loss is not about deprivation. You'll lose weight on a Gluten-Free diet IF you do it the right way. If you do it the wrong way, those extra pounds will cling to your hips, stomach and thighs. And in fact, you can gain weight if you get lazy in your food choices.

And remember, even at your current weight, there is nothing wrong with you. You are perfect just the way you are.

Losing weight is about embracing the concepts of patience and discipline. In my teens, 20's and 30's I worked out excessively. I cared only about how I looked, not about how healthy I was. By my 40's I had burned out my knees by teaching up to 5 aerobic classes per day (in my 20's), running long distances and cycling long distance. I stopped exercising altogether and gained over 60 lbs. I was so fed up with exercise that I did very little and spent more time recipe testing and wine tasting for my cookbooks. Now in my 50's I've finally learned the magic of patience and discipline as it relates to my health and weight. Or said another way, I've restored the integrity in this aspect of my life. I eat a healthy, Gluten-Free diet, walk only 3 miles on a regular basis and drink wine moderately. I sample my recipes (instead of devouring the dishes) and I assess wines on a regular basis. I don't overindulge. My cholesterol is normal. I have low blood pressure and take no medications whatsoever.

This lifestyle is about reaching a weight for overall health and to prevent and/or control diseases and conditions. When overweight, we put ourselves at risk of developing serious health issues, including heart disease, high blood pressure, type 2 diabetes, gallstones, breathing problems, cancers, sleep apnea, osteoarthritis, fatty liver disease, kidney disease, arthritis, to name but a few.

The Gluten-Free lifestyle should be utilized to reach and maintain a healthy weight.

Chapter 1: What is Gluten?

Gluten is a protein found in wheat, barley, and rye. It is a composite created when two proteins (glutenin and gliadin) are mixed with water and form hydrogen bonds, allowing them to form a sturdy network. It is this ability that has made gluten-containing grains preferable for baking bread and making pasta. Gluten creates structure. It allows bread to hold its shape, absorb moisture and become more elastic. It gives pasta that wonderful al dente texture. Gluten is readily used in soups, sauces, spices, gravies, and thickeners, and even in beer and liquor.

Oats are Gluten-Free, but can be gluten contaminated. Most commercial oats are processed in facilities that also process wheat, barley, and rye. So if you have Celiac disease or are highly sensitive to gluten, refrain from eating oats, unless you know they are free from contamination.

Any food that is but one ingredient cannot have gluten in it. Single ingredient products are good for us. Fruits, vegetables, meat, poultry and fish are healthy, as are lentils, nuts, corn, and rice. Even chocolate, wine and dairy products can be nutritional, when consumed in moderation.

There are distinctions to be made between Celiac disease, wheat allergies and gluten intolerance and sensitivity.

If you believe you may suffer from one of these conditions, it's extremely important to consult your doctor.

What's important to know is that the wheat we consume today and the super rate in which we incorporate wheat into our diet through a plethora of products is not the same wheat consumed by our ancestors. Today's wheat is considered by many to be a Frankenstein version of the original grain.

There are 3 cultivated wheat species. They are Diplois, Diploid and Tetrapoid. Wheat varieties within each species have varying levels of the gluten proteins called gliadin and glutenin. Gliadin is the soluble element in gluten; glutenin is the insoluble element.

Those suffering from Celiac disease or gluten-intolerance are reacting to gliadin protein. Gliadin causes an inflammatory reaction as it comes into contact with the wall of the small intestine. This low-grade inflammation may go undetected for years before symptoms become obvious. This can cause a slow destruction of the healthy living tissues within the small intestine. Over time gliadin intolerance creates significant stress on the immune system.

Our ancestors, found in the Great Rift Valley of Africa about 2.6 million years ago, consumed a wild species of wheat called Einkorn. Einkorn (of the Diplois species) is non-genetically altered with 14 chromosomes of gliadin.

In the 1950's scientists began crossbreeding and hybridizing wheat to make it hardier, shorter, and able to resist pests and diseases. As crop rotation was applied to long cultivated land, along with the use of fertilizers, yields of wheat increased. Wheat was required to feed larger populations of people across the globe. What we now know is that this morphing of wheat from its ancient form to its present version also introduced compounds believed to be unfriendly to the human digestive system.

Today's wheat variety (called bread or common wheat and part of the Diploid species) is the most widely grown and used for the production of almost all commercial wheat products today. Common wheat has strong and elastic gluten that enables its dough to trap carbon dioxide during leavening and is therefore beneficial in the making of baked products like bread. The issue is that common wheat has a grand total of 42 chromosomes of gliadin -- not 14 like its ancestral version.

Durum wheat (part of the Tetrapoid species) is used for making pasta and contains 28 chromosomes of gliadin.

Durum and Bread wheat contain more than double and triple the amount of the protein gliadin as found in the ancient grain

Einkorn. These hybridized and crossbred varieties are often referred to as 'super glutens' or 'Frankenwheats.'

Why should we care about the level of the protein gliadin in our breads and pastas? The reason is that high levels of gliadin are believed to trigger inflammation in the body. Inflammation then triggers insulin resistance, causing an increase in the appetite, gradual weight gain, and ultimately diabetes.

Research shows that super gluten wheat raises blood sugar levels, causing immunoreactive problems, inhibits the absorption of important minerals, and aggravates our intestines. These wheat are now believed by many scientists and experts to contribute to obesity, diabetes, heart disease, cancer, dementia, depression and an excess of other illnesses.

(Keep in mind that there are researchers, scientists, physicians and experts on the other side of the argument who will adamantly argue that wheat does not lead to these health conditions. They believe that if you are not suffering from Celiac disease or gluten sensitivity, then removing it from the diet is unnecessary and even ludicrous.)

No source of Frankenwheat — not newly sprouted or in baked bread, pasta or pastries -- is good for us.

Other Grains with Gliadin Structures

Rye and barley share similar gliadin structures to wheat.

There is much controversy over corn. In relation to Celiac disease, corn has not been studied to the same extent as wheat. But thus far studies show that corn proteins on the celiac intestine are safe.

Chapter 2: Secrets to the Gluten-Free Lifestyle

Unlike a fad diet made up of rules, such as eliminating all fat or counting calories, the Gluten-Free lifestyle is exactly that -- a lifestyle choice. The only rule is to eliminate or substitute foods containing gluten. There are, however, choices you can make to ensure you are pursuing this lifestyle in a healthy way, all the while losing weight. There are also secrets, tips and ideas to utilize along the way to lose and maintain a comfortable weight

Secret 1: Manage Your Stressors

One of the most important ways to support weight loss is to create a stress free or stress reduced life. This can be done by incorporating activities, such as yoga and meditation and distances ourselves from those who have a negative impact on you. You can always love people from a distance.

When we experience stress or sudden danger, our brain signals our body to turn out a hormone called cortisol.

Cortisol is a steroid hormone secreted by the adrenal glands. Its primary functions are to increase blood sugar through gluconeogenesis, suppress the immune system, and aid the metabolism of fat, protein, and carbohydrate.

When experiencing stress, cortisol sends a message throughout the body to mobilize us for a life-saving response. It gives us a burst of increased energy, heightened memory function, and a lower sensitivity to pain. Our heart races and we become highly attentive. Vigilant. Our metabolism shifts. Energy is made rapidly available to our muscles, preparing them for action. When the emergency subsides, the cortisol acts as its own shut-off signal. It is important for the body to return to normal.

Cortisol is a positive response system when we experience sudden stress or danger. But it can also have a negative effect on us if our stress is chronic.

If our life is full of stressors we can experience what is referred to as chronic stress. With chronic stress, our body moves to code red and we experience anxiety, vigilance, and hyper-alertness and even anxiety attacks continuously. When we are seized by chronic stress, the cortisol signal does not shut off. The prolonged release of cortisol results in significant physiological changes. Some of these are impaired cognitive performance, suppressed thyroid function, blood sugar imbalances such as hyperglycemia, decreased bone density, decreased muscle tissue, high blood pressure, lowered immunity and inflammatory responses in the body, and slowing down healing.

And in the context of this book, chronic stress leads to abdominal fat. Too much abdominal fat leads to health problems, such as heart attacks, strokes, high levels of bad cholesterol (LDL) and the development of metabolic syndrome. Metabolic syndrome is a group of cardiac risk factors like type 2 diabetes and cardiovascular disease.

When experiencing stress we also reach for comfort foods. Comfort foods are made up of taste sensations or what are also known as our survival mechanisms. During stressful situations, food can provide us with a sense of comfort, even if this moment is fleeting.

We eat to stay alive. Our survival mechanisms are the taste sensations of sweetness, sourness, saltiness, and bitterness (and some might say umami (depth of flavor) and fattiness. Our survival mechanisms are developed when we were still in the mother's womb. So at the moment of birth we have an instinctive craving for these taste sensations. We taste mother's milk for the first time, experience its sweetness and crave more, thus staying alive. We crave saltiness, which keeps our body hydrated. This is so our body does not dehydrate, thus causing death. We crave sourness, as foods with a sour taste sensation like citrus fruits, provides vitamins like vitamin C to thwart off diseases, such as scurvy. We also can sense foods that have soured, like soured milk, that could make us sick and therefore put us in harm's way. And we crave bitterness. Foods with bitterness like walnuts, provide vitamins and minerals that also ward off cancers and other illnesses.

Stress causes us to desire and even instinctively crave for our survival mechanisms, the taste sensations that make up delicious comfort foods!

Said another way, one of the primary secrets to succeeding at losing weight within the Gluten-Free lifestyle is to reduce and even eliminate all the circumstances in your life causing you stress.

Secret 2: Eat in a Healthy Way

The Gluten-Free lifestyle for weight loss supports the notion of eating single ingredient foods – fruits, vegetables, fish, poultry and lean meats. It embodies the philosophy of staying away from Gluten-Free boxed and processed foods that are usually high in calories, sugar, fat and preservatives. It means focusing on and eating fruits and vegetables and gluten-free grains that do not stimulate the appetite or raise your blood sugar levels. And it means consuming products, such as dairy, chocolate and wine or with saturated fat in moderation. Eating low glycemic foods ultimately leads to gradual weight loss over time. Going Gluten-Free is by no means a crash diet.

According to a study by researchers at Dalhousie University in Halifax, Canada, published in the Canadian Journal of Dietetic Practice and Research in 2008, Gluten-Free products are a $4.2 billion dollar enterprise in the United States; $90-million in Canada.

This study also revealed that Gluten-Free products are 242% more expensive than their regular counterparts, and 455% pricier in some cases.

This is certainly true for me. I pay over $6.00 for a loaf artisan Gluten-Free bread. But I eat so little bread that it's worth the investment.

"Being gluten-free is a good thing, but eating gluten-free processed foods is not a good thing," says Dr. William Davis, author of the best-selling book Wheat Belly: Lose the Wheat, Lose the Weight and Find Your Path Back to Health and US cardiologist. (CTVNews.ca)

Eating too much Gluten-Free processed food (what I call gluten-free junk food) like Gluten-Free cookies, cakes and processed food has a high glycemic load on your system. Just because it is Gluten-Free, doesn't mean it is healthy. Gluten-Free cakes and cookies are still cakes and cookies! I know I am repeating myself. Vegetables, fruits, beans, nuts and seeds and lean animal protein are all Gluten Free. Eat them. They should be the primary source of your diet.

"We don't want to replace one problem with other problems," says Dr. Davis. "Foods that raise your blood sugar sky-high, make your tummy grow, give you hyper-tension, dementia, cancer and heart disease." (CTVNews.ca)

Secret 3: One Happy Day Per Week

My ex-husband used to own and operate a chain of fitness centers throughout the 1980's and 90's. The fitness centers catered to body builders and so I was immersed in that scene and had my own body building trainer. I also interviewed body builders about their diets for body building magazines. I learned about a secret that body builders utilize throughout the year to help them lose weight. It's called the 'fat loading day.' The fat loading day should take place about once per week or once every two weeks when you're first starting your Gluten-Free journey. On that day you eat all the fatty foods you like, as long as they are Gluten-Free. The theory is that the increase in fat and calories into the body shocks the metabolism. This process speeds up the metabolism, which of course increases weight loss. The key to this secret, however, is to maintain a disciplined exercise routine. Refrain from fat loading days if you are not committed to regular exercise.

Secret 4: Low Glycemic Foods

On a regular basis it is important to eat foods low on the glycemic index. The glycemic index was originally designed to support diabetics in controlling their blood sugar levels. What helps to control blood sugar has also proven to support weight loss.

Foods on the glycemic index are scored, ranging on a scale from 0 to 100 based on the increase of the blood sugar level. High G-I foods (ranging 70 and higher) include white foods like rice, pasta, bread, bagels, potatoes, along with sugar-sweetened beverages (to name a few).

Medium-GI foods (56 to 69) include fruits like bananas and grapes, along with corn on the cob, spaghetti and ice cream.

Low-GI foods (55 and under) include peanuts, peas, carrots, kidney beans, hummus, skim milk and most fruits.

Secret 5: Stimulate Your Metabolism

Dr. William Davis, M.D. believes that going Gluten-Free tends to decrease your cravings and appetite overall, that is, after your initial cravings for wheat-based foods has subsided. I don't believe in calorie counting. Being Gluten-Free should be a lifestyle change, not an obsessive diet.

Be sure to also fluctuate your calorie count from one day to the next. This keeps the metabolism stimulated (rather than complacent), thus keeping you from plateauing in your weight loss.

Secret 6: Eat more vegetables, fruits and nuts

Remember, it isn't just the wheat carbs that increase our cravings and appetite. It's high glycemic foods, in general. Limit your high-carb foods. Eat them occasionally. Did you know that 2 slices of whole grain bread contains about 138 calories? You get the same amount of fiber in 24 almonds (also 138 calories).

Secret 7: Make Sure It's Gluten-Free

Many people believe they are Gluten-Free when they are not. It's important to watch out for the hidden sources of gluten. Read the last chapter on reading labels.

Secret 8: Eat Organic, Free Range, Grass-Fed

My husband and I fundamentally eat an organic, vegetarian-based, Gluten-Free diet when at home. It doesn't have to be a difficult life-style to maintain if you enjoy dining out.

One of the best ways to ensure products are organic is to eat local when possible and visit your local farms. I'm fortunate to be living in the heart of farm country where I can obtain local, fresh and organic products from the farmers and from our local, Saturday farmer's market. Organic farmers care about their impact on soil life and fertility, water systems and conservation, air quality and the sustainability of the local and big picture eco-system.

(Not all organic designations are legitimate. That's why I advocate that you eat local and visit farms!)

I have pernicious anemia and so require sufficient doses of vitamin B-12 through food, vitamins and shots. Every once in a while I crave beef. The fact is beef contains high quality protein and nutrients like Creatine and Carnosine, which are important for our muscles and brain.

We have a hefty beef farming industry in our community. And in our community there is much controversy over corn-fed versus grass-fed beef. One of my best friends is a beef farmer who advocates that there is nothing wrong with GMO corn fed cows. It is one of the few issues we choose to disagree on. The choice is yours.

I believe that the way cows are fed has a major effect on the quality and nutritional value of the beef. Many scientists agree. Historically, cows ate grass. This affects their digestive track, PH levels and the fatty acid composition of the meat.

Studies show that grass-fed beef is less in total saturated and monounsaturated fats. There are 3 main types of saturated fat found in red meat. They are: stearic acid, palmitic acid, and mystristic acid. Grass-fed beef consistently contains higher proportion of stearic acid, which does not raise blood cholesterol levels.

Grass-fed beef is also 5-times higher in Omega-3's and has 2 to 3 times as much conjugated linoleic acid (CLA). CLA is a fatty acid associated with reduced body fat and exhibits potent antioxidant activity. Research reveals that CLA might also protect us from heart disease, diabetes and cancer.

Grass-fed beef is also lower in calories and high in Vitamin A, Vitamin E and micronutrients like potassium, iron, zinc, phosphorus and sodium.

If at all possible, buy beef directly from the farmer where you can witness first hand how the animals live and are treated.

Secret 9: Exercise

Exercising is key to any weight loss program. Moderate exercise performed three times per week will help you feel better, give you more energy and help you live longer. The health benefits of regular exercise cannot be ignored.

Along with pursuing a Gluten-Free lifestyle, regular exercise will help prevent further weight gain and support you in maintaining your weight loss. Exercise makes the body burn calories. It's that simple. The more intense the exercise, the more calories you'll burn.

Exercise also helps to combat health conditions and diseases. It boosts your high-density lipoprotein (HDL or good cholesterol and decreases unhealthy triglycerides. This keeps your blood flowing smoothly, thus decreasing your risk of cardiovascular disease. Regular exercise also helps to reduce your risk of a stroke, metabolic syndrome, type 2 diabetes, depression, cancers, and arthritis.

Feeling low? Try exercise! A brisk 30-minute walk three times per week stimulates brain chemicals that leave you feeling happier and more relaxed.

Most importantly, exercise boosts energy. Exercise delivers oxygen and nutrients to your muscles and tissues, thus helping your lungs and heart work more efficiently.

Chapter 3: How Does Gluten Affect Your Health?

It may be true that only about 1 percent of Americans need to be Gluten-Free because of the autoimmune disorder called Celiac Disease.

Some scientists, experts and doctors say that moving to a Gluten-Free lifestyle won't give you any additional nutritional or health benefits and will not help you lose weight.

We are all entitled to our opinions, even the expert ones.

Other research has shown that the average person consumes about 55 pounds of wheat products each year. More physicians like Dr. William Davis, MD, (author of the best-selling book called Wheat Belly), neurologists like Dr. David Perlmutter (author of the best-selling book called Grain Brain) and naturopathic doctors, such as Peter Glidden (advocate and speaker) believe that a wheat, rye and barley-free diet is a healthy lifestyle choice for everyone. It can help us heal our body, mind, and spirit and help us shed unwanted weight.

Dr. Glidden advocates that gluten is a difficult protein for the body to digest. Difficult for every human body. The reason is that protein (despite its source) has long chains of amino acids that are linked together through chemical bonds. There are 12 amino acids, which are essential nutrients that our body needs to import on a daily basis.

Our stomach is supposed to break the chemical bonds, liberating the free amino acids to be chewed and digested and absorbed. The source of the protein distinguishes its structure. The structure of protein can be vastly different from one source or ingredient to another. Herein lies the issue. The chemical bond in wheat, barley, and rye is difficult for the human stomach to digest.

It is through the small intestines that all the nutrition from food is absorbed. Our small intestines contain millions of villi. On top of the villi are thousands of microvilli. In our intestinal track there are billions of tissues designed to absorb nutrients. It's the job of the villi to stick onto a molecule of digested food and suck the nutrients from it and put it into the blood stream. The body cannot utilize nutrients until they are digested and absorbed by the bloodstream.

The chemical bonds of wheat, barley, and rye are difficult to break. When you eat these products, the protein is left undigested. An undigested protein tumbling through the intestinal track acts like a live wire, zapping and destroying the villi. It is the job of the villi to absorb nutrients. So if the villi are destroyed, the body is unable to absorb nutrients. The result is mal-absorption, which is the primary cause of most chronic diseases.

Living a Gluten-Free lifestyle to lose weight is the first benefit. But this lifestyle change has other benefits, as well. Here are a few:

Improved Digestion
The second benefit of a Gluten-Free style is that it greatly maintains and improves the digestive system. A lot of people who have undertaken a Gluten-Free lifestyle noticed a mild to drastic change in terms of their digestion in a short period of time. They have said that there has been a noticeable improvement in bowel movements and a great reduction in indigestion. There is also a significant decrease in bloating and cramps, which is a definite plus for women.

Reduced Joint Inflammation
The third benefit of a Gluten-Free lifestyle is that it reduces inflammation in various tissues in the body. People who are highly sensitive and allergic to gluten usually experience episodes of pain in joints, muscles, and legs. People who also experience inflammation on the skin such as Dermatitis, Eczema, or Dermatitis Herpetiformis will reap some benefits from a Gluten-Free lifestyle, as well.

My husband has noticed that he experiences less pain in his hips and knees.

Increased Energy Levels

The fourth benefit of a Gluten-Free lifestyle is that it improves energy levels especially in those people who suffer from Celiac Disease, sensitivity or intolerance to gluten. It has been reported that people who consume too much gluten experience a lot of tiredness and weakness. Gluten-related fatigue can be disruptive and even debilitating.

Researches are still not entirely clear what causes fatigue in those with Celiac Disease or gluten-intolerance. But fatigue is recognized as one of the top symptoms. One speculation is that fatigue is caused by malnutrition or anemia.

While still not scientifically proven, gluten ingestion plays a direct role in sleep problems for people with Celiac Disease and gluten sensitivity. Dr. Rodney Ford, a New Zealand pediatrician and author of *The Gluten Syndrome*, believes that a gluten diet affects the brain and neurological tissue directly. This causes symptoms. However, there is no direct research revealing this fact.

Reducing one's gluten intake or simply going Gluten-Free will help to support your getting those energy levels pumping.

Improved Blood-Sugar Levels
The fifth benefit is that going Gluten-Free will help keep your blood sugar levels at bay. Food products with gluten are usually accompanied by significant sugar. So switching to a lifestyle made up of the consumption of more single ingredients like fruits and vegetables and foods that do not contain gluten will help you to control your blood sugar and fat intake.

Chapter 4: How Does Gluten Make You Fat?

As we know, gluten is a protein found in wheat, barley and rye. We consume far more wheat than the other grains. Wheat eaters consume an average of 400 extra calories per day, which equals about 42 pounds of additional weight gain over time.

This is not surprising, given our addiction to bread and pasta!

Frankenwheat (dwarfed and hybridized), discussed earlier, has a high glycemic index, which contributes to stored belly fat, which can trigger insulin resistance, causing weight gain. It also makes for a fatty liver, leading to obesity, pre-diabetes, diabetes and about 44 other conditions like autoimmune diseases, irritable bowel, reflux, cancer, depression, osteoporosis and more.

Frankenwheat also contains a super starch called amylopectin A, which is super fattening. When wheat is consumed, the body ingests a huge helping of a blood sugar-spiking carbohydrate called amylopectin-A. To move the sugars from the wheat into your cells where they can be used for energy - or stored as fat, the pancreas responds by releasing insulin. After consuming food, the higher the blood sugar, the greater the insulin release, the more fat is deposited in the abdominal area. This is called visceral fat.

When visceral fat builds up, it floods the body with toxins and inflammatory signals that cause muscle to stop responding to a proportional amount of insulin.

In turn the pancreas produces more insulin to help metabolize the carbohydrates consumed. After years of putting the body through this high-blood sugar, high-insulin cycle, it acquires visceral fat. Dr. William Davis, MD, refers to this visceral fat as the "wheat belly." The surge of glucose and insulin and drop in blood sugar is what makes us hungry 2 hours later.

Unlike other grains, wheat is also super addictive. In fact, its effect on the brain is equal to that of opiate drugs. Researchers at the National Institutes of Health found that gluten polypeptides penetrate blood-brain barriers. Once entered in the brain, wheat compounds bind to the brain's morphine receptors (the same receptors to which opiate drugs bind), thus producing a sense of euphoria.

The Beer Belly

Is the wheat belly and the beer belly one and the same?

I am a wine and food journalist and author by trade. I've been around a lot of alcohol and alcohol consumers over the past 22 years. Have you ever wondered why there is no such term as "wine belly?" Why do we call it a beer belly or beer gut?

Some doctors and scientists believe the beer belly derives from the extra caloric intake from alcohol. This is true. Alcohol consumption also stimulates the appetite and we tend to eat more when consuming wine or beer. It's also true that alcohol slows the metabolism, thus adding extra calories. And when we drink alcohol, we tend to relax more and exert less. In other words, we don't burn off the additional calories consumed.

But I personally believe there's more to it. Chronic beer drinkers tend to have an identifiable roundness and bloat to their bellies. Could it be symptoms of brewed Frankenwheat?

Those with Celiac Disease or gluten intolerance cannot drink beer. And those with gluten sensitivities also experience symptoms from the gluten in this beverage. When my brother Jay drinks beer his ankles swell. I become excessively bloated.

I personally think wheat eaters that also love beer can suffer from the classic 'beer belly.'

Chapter 5: Another Secret. Avoid Some Gluten-Free Foods

Just because a grain is Gluten-Free does not mean you should go hog-wild in consuming it. There are Gluten-Free grains that can actually cause you to gain weight if you eat them too often. Millet and whole grain cornmeal are examples.

Millet

Originating in China, this particular grain can be used as a substitute for rice-based recipes; even risotto or polenta as it develops a creamy based texture.

It is high in B vitamins and fiber and it provides alkalizing benefits to the body. In terms of taste, Millet has a sugary yet nutty flavor. This particular grain is digestible and only a few people are known to be allergic to it. Millet also prevents constipation by making sure the colon is well hydrated. Since Millet is considered as a smart carb, it basically contains an immense amount of fiber and low plain sugars, which helps in keeping the blood sugar levels of the body healthy and in tip-top shape.

BUT, do not over indulge in eating millet if you want to lose weight. Millet contains goitrogen, which increases after cooking. Goitrogen is believed to suppress thyroid activity and can lead to depression, difficulty in losing weight, and fatigue.

Whole Grain Cornmeal

While whole grain cornmeal contains a lot of vitamins and minerals such as iron, phosphorus, magnesium, zinc, and vitamin B-6, it is also high in calories. So eat it sparingly if you want to lose weight through the Gluten-Free lifestyle. One cup of cornmeal has 500 calories! According to research, cornmeal is said to be great in helping improve digestion, reduce high blood pressure, and lessen the risk of acquiring heart disease, gallstones, etc.

Gluten-Free Granola

Be wary of Gluten-Free granola. While using Gluten-Free grains, it may also be high in calories and contain hydrogenated fats because they extend shelf life and make the grains softer. Granola usually contains nuts and seeds, which help to spike the fat content as well. The sugar content whether its sugar, honey or maple can also be high, which sends the blood sugar out of whack and contributes toward weight gain.

Gluten-Free Bread

Just because the package says "Gluten-Free" does not mean the item is good for you. Some Gluten-Free breads are high in saturated fat. Lard is often used in making Gluten-Free breads stay moist. Two slices can be as much as 240 calories.

Gluten-Free Frozen Pizza

Just like breads, Gluten-Free pre-made and frozen pizzas can have as much fat as a take-out cheeseburger. I've seen calories as high as 500 for a mini-sized pizza. Make your own. Once you've found the Gluten-Free All-Purpose Flour blend that you enjoy, pizza dough can be super easy to make.

Gluten-Free Short Bread Cookies

Short bread cookies are high in fat, whether they are Gluten-Free or not. Stay away from them or only eat them occasionally.

Cream-Based Soups

Cream-based soups are made with a white roux, consisting of flour, butter and milk or cream. Gluten-Free versions use Gluten-Free flour, but also contain butter and cream. Make your own cream-based soups by substituting the cream for fat-free condensed milk or stock-based versions. In my community I can buy fat-free cream. It's a tasty base in homemade cream-based soups.

Ice Cream

Some commercial ice creams use wheat as a thickening agent. So, be sure to check before consuming it. Also, be careful of blended ice cream flavors as they often contain gluten, as well, such as chocolate chip cookie dough.

Some of the most popular Gluten-Free ice cream brands include Ben and Jerry's, Breyer's Ice Cream, Dove Ice Cream, Haagen-Dazs, Talenti, Turkey Hill Dairy and So Delicious.

Other Foods to Avoid

Refined Sugar (see next chapter)

Soy Sauce:

Stay away from Chinese soy sauce, which contains wheat. Tamari-based soy sauce, usually served with Japanese food, is mostly produced without wheat. Some brands, however, might contain wheat, so be careful if you suffer from Celiac Disease or you are gluten-intolerant. Kikkoman is my favorite brand.

Sausages and Luncheon Meats

Wheat flour is often used as bulking filler in processed meats and sausages. Hunt for Gluten-Free versions.

Salad Dressings

Wheat flour is often used as a thickening agent in cream and oil based dressings. Check out the ingredient list on the brand's website or make your own.

Pre-made Sauces and Gravies

Like salad dressings, premade sauces and gravies or packages of dried versions usually contain wheat flour used as a thickening agent.

Vitamins

Yes, vitamins may contain gluten and it probably won't be listed on the bottle. Check with the manufacturer.

Tortilla Chips

We think tortilla chips made with corn flour are automatically Gluten-Free. This may not be the case. Check with the brand's website or buy only tortilla chips that are marked as 'Gluten-Free' on the bag.

Ketchup

While some ketchup can contain gluten, Heinz does not. It is Gluten-Free.

Candy

Jellybeans and licorice contain gluten and 'Gluten-Free' usually does not appear on the packaging.

Chapter 6: Gluten-Free Secrets and Tips

The Best Gluten-Free All-Purpose Flour Blend

Find the best (for you) all-purpose flour blend. Once you've found a recipe or brand of Gluten-Free flour blend, cooking G-Free will be easy.

How to Reduce Fat While Cooking:

We often fry foods with oil because we've been conditioned to do so. When foods are being served individually such as shrimp over noodles, then frying adds flavor and a crispy texture. But there are lots of places where water can replace oil in cooking to reduce the over all fat content of a dish. When I'm making chicken stroganoff or Sheppard's pie or cabbage rolls or meat sauce for spaghetti, I sauté the onion, garlic, mushrooms, celery and spinach and the meat in water. When many ingredients are being incorporated, the oil used for sautéing will add only minimal flavor. So, reduce the over all fat content of the dish by replacing oil with water.

Bring your own Gluten-Free Soy Sauce to Japanese and Chinese Restaurants: When eating sushi, avoid any rolls with tempura. Tempura is the deep dried coating on vegetables and shrimp. It is often incorporated into sushi rolls. Tempura is made with panko crumbs, which are made with wheat. You can pick a plethora of sushi items on the menu that are tempura free.

Make Your Own Panko Crumbs

Make your own panko crumbs for coating chicken, fish and shrimp. Place about 3 cups of Gluten-Free Rice Chex Cereal in a plastic lunch bag. Use a rolling pin to crush the cereal to coarse flakes. You can add Gluten-Free All-Purpose flour to help with the cereal stick to the foods and add your own seasonings.

The Secrets to Making Perfect Gluten-Free Spaghetti and Meatballs

When I started living a Gluten-Free lifestyle, I resented that I had to give up spaghetti and meatballs. This is no longer the case.

I've discovered the secrets to making perfect Gluten-Free spaghetti and meatballs.

Secret #1: IT STARTS WITH THE SAUCE: I operate a cooking club. We held a blind tasting of different brands of canned tomatoes, including the authentic Italian (coded) Marzano brand which was marked as double the price. Alta Cucina tomatoes from California (with no preservatives) came first in the blind tasting. This brand produces superior tasting tomatoes with excellent color, texture and flavor. So, the secret is to choose fresh tomatoes over canned ones. But if you have no choice, choose highly flavorful canned tomatoes like Alta Cucina.

Secret #2: THE NOODLE: The secret, I believe, is to ensure your Gluten-Free pasta is made from corn flour or from a mixture of more corn flour (first) than rice flour combined. Dried pastas that list rice flour as the first ingredient tend to quickly lose their al dente texture and become graining and mushy. I've tried several brands and am always disappointed.

I recently found Barilla Gluten-Free Spaghetti. This brand also produces other pasta shapes, as well. I love it. It is close in texture and taste to classic wheat-based pasta.

Pasta made with only corn flour also retain their lovely al dente texture.

So the secret is to make sure the dried pasta lists corn flour as the first ingredient.

Secret #3: THE COOKING PROCESS: When cooking wheat-based spaghetti you don't rinse the noodles. The point is for the starch to grab onto the sauce. Not so with Gluten-Free pasta. To make perfect Gluten-Free pasta, it's all about the size of the pot, the fanning of the noodles, the rolling boil, the foaming pasta water, the changing color of the pasta, and then the rinsing. Fan the noodles out on both ends before putting them into the water. Be sure to stir them constantly, bringing them up and out of the water to loosen them from each other. Keep the water rolling. Test for doneness. Be sure to rinse them.

Secret #4: THE MEATBALLS: There are a few secrets to producing perfect Gluten-Free meatballs. The first tip is to be extra careful when working with any ground meat. Watch for cross contamination. Work with one food item at a time, such as the ground meat, then scrub your cutting board with extremely hot water, strong detergent and a good brush. I also like to spray my board with a mixture of peroxide and water. Then wash your hands before moving onto another food item.

Older cutting boards, especially plastic ones, often have deep and shallow scratches and grooves from past use. These grooves act as a breeding ground for bacterial. If your guests get sick from your meatballs, they are hardly perfect. So, cleanliness and diligence are an important technique to utilize.

The secret is to make sure the meatballs hold together and don't crumble. You can do this by ensuring all the air is removed from the raw flesh. In other words, abuse your meat. I know this is contrary to what you normally hear, but I obtained this secret from a friend of mine who is a Chef de Cuisine, the highest rank one can obtain in Canada in the culinary industry.

The next secret is to ensure your meatballs cook evenly. So use a small ice cream scoop or melon baller to make them all the same size. Wet your hands with cool water when shaping the meatballs to help prevent sticking.

Next? Boil the meat balls before baking or grilling them. Boil the balls until they float. This helps to keep them in one piece and ensures they are cooked.

The next secret? Make your meatballs in different shapes. This gives the meatballs a more homemade feel and adds variety to the eyes. Try flattening them slightly or making them oblong.

Here's a recipe I make.

Traditional Italian Gluten-Free Meatballs

Serves 6

1 pound of ground veal

1 pound of ground pork

1 pound of ground beef

½-cup finely chopped yellow onion

½-cup freshly grated Parmigiano-Reggiano

1 clove garlic, minced

2 tablespoons dried oregano

2 tablespoons chopped fresh parsley

1 teaspoon salt

½ teaspoon freshly ground black pepper

1 egg, beaten

1 tablespoon extra virgin olive oil

¼-cup Gluten-Free breadcrumbs*

Be sure to add spinach, onions and mushrooms to your sauce so that you can create a spaghetti sauce loaded in B-complex vitamins!

Take your favorite 1 loaf of any type of gluten-free bread. Break into small pieces and place on a baking sheet. Bake in a 400-degree F oven until brown and crisp (about 10 minutes). Remove from the oven and place in a food processor. Grind them into fine crumbs. Place all ingredients into a bowl. Mix well with your hands. Squeeze air out of mixture, throwing it back onto the bowl. Refrigerate for one hour to let mixture rest and let flavors come together. Make balls, about one ounce of meat, by rolling tightly to remove any air. Line baking tray with parchment paper. Preheat oven to 350 F. In large pot of boiling water, par cook meat balls until they float, about two minutes. Transfer meatballs to baking tray. Transfer to the oven and bake for 15 minutes or until brown. Serve with fresh pasta in favorite tomato sauce.

Secret #5: THE CHEESE: If you garnish your spaghetti and meatballs with cheese, be sure to freshly grate Parmigiano-Reggiano. Do not waste your hard-earned money on already grated cheese that has dried out and lost most of its flavor. And stick to the real deal – Parmigiano-Reggiano. Avoid North American versions of this authentic cheese.

Secret #6: USE FRESH HERBS: While you can add fresh herbs to the sauce during the cooking process, be sure to add chopped fresh herbs as a garnish. Nothing is tastier than chopped fresh basil and a drizzle of olive oil over the cheese on spaghetti sauce.

Secret #7: THE WINE: This is a classic Italian dish deserving of a quality glass of Italian wine. Remember tomato sauce made from fresh tomatoes and even canned tomatoes has refreshing acidity that resembles the real fruit. So, choose an Italian red wine with enough acidity to match. Chianti Classico Reserva. While this is a rustic dish, the time it takes to prepare it demands a quality wine for celebration.

Chapter 7: Gluten-Free Grains that Support Weight Loss

A study published in the American Journal of Clinical Nutrition underscores the importance of choosing whole grains such as brown rice rather than refined grains, i.e., white rice, to maintain a healthy body weight. In this Harvard Medical School / Brigham and Women's Hospital study, which collected data on over 74,000 female nurses aged 38-63 years over a 12 year period, weight gain was associated with the intake of refined-grain foods. It revealed that women who consumed more whole grains were 49% less likely to gain weight compared to those eating foods made from refined grains.

The Gluten-Free diet requires the complete elimination of all wheat, rye and barley products.

Gluten-Free replacements for cereals and baking mixes are often made up of a combination of cornstarch, potato starch, tapioca starch and/or white rice flour. The nutrient composition of these ingredients falls short in comparison to those provided by whole grains.

That's why it is important for you to incorporate Gluten-Free whole grains into your diet on a daily basis. Without whole grains, you can become deficient in important minerals, vitamins, fiber, calcium, and iron.

Store whole grains in airtight containers. Store them for no longer than a year in a cool, dark place. Millet should be consumed within 2 to 3 months. Whole grain flours will last up to 6 months or in the freezer for up to a year.

When cooking whole grains, remember that they double or triple in size once cooked. For flavoring add broths, stocks, juice or milk in place of water. Before cooking grains, be sure to rinse them first. Bring the liquid to a boil and then reduce to simmer. You need not stir the grains. Once the grains absorb the liquid and are tender, remove them from the heat and let them sit for about 5 minutes.

Cook more than you need and store the extra cooked grains in the freezer.

In undertaking the Gluten-Free lifestyle, there are whole grains that support weight loss and others that sabotage it.

Buckwheat

Despite its name, buckwheat is not wheat. In fact, it isn't a grain at all. It's a fruit seed of a plant that is related to rhubarb. These grain-like seeds have a unique triangular shape and are the same size as wheat kernels. Buckwheat can be ground into flour and substitute other wheat, rye, barley and oats in recipes.

If you are embracing the Gluten-Free lifestyle, then you'll want to also embrace this fruit! It is fat free, low in calories, fills you up faster, facilitates proper digestion, builds lean muscle mass and suppresses the appetite. What more can you ask for in a seed?

Most importantly, buckwheat is low on the glycemic index, thus supporting weight loss by releasing energy slowly and controlling your blood sugar level.

Buckwheat contains a medicinal chemical that strengthens capillary walls and reduces hemorrhage, thus lowering the risk of fatal strokes and heart attacks in people with high blood pressure and diabetes. It improves micro vascular integrity and circulation in diabetics, thus preventing the damage of nerves and muscle cells and loss of kidney function.

As a good source of magnesium, Buckwheat helps to improve blood pressure by relaxing the blood vessels. As a rich source of B vitamins (niacin, folate and B6), this seed contributes toward our cardiovascular health. These vitamins enhance blood vessel strength and bad cholesterol removal. Buckwheat's iron, magnesium, phosphorus, copper and manganese help to improve blood oxygenation. It contains these high quality proteins, which remove the plaque forming triglycerides and low-density lipoproteins (LDL). Thus buckwheat is highly beneficial for all of us, especially those with weak heart functions and other cardiovascular problems.

Buckwheat contains D-chiro-Inositol. This is a compound that is deficient in type II diabetic patients and is required for proper conduction of insulin for controlling and treating type II diabetes.

Because it is composed of cellulose, buckwheat removes toxins from the body, acting as a cleansing ingredient. And as an insoluble fiber, Buckwheat helps to prevent gallstones. It speeds up the removal of food through the intestines, increases insulin sensitivity but lowers the secretion of bile acids and blood sugar.

A diet rich in Buckwheat can also help reduce the risk of breast cancer. Its antioxidant properties are also beneficial for women during and after menopause, thus protecting against the risk of breast cancer and other forms of cancers related to hormones.

Buckwheat has an abundance of other health benefits, as well. It strengthens bones by facilitating the absorption of calcium. It contains tryptophan to influence our mood and helps to prevent depression and strengthens our immune system against flu and the common cold.

The secret to implementing buckwheat for weight loss is to eat it partially raw. When it is cooked buckwheat loses its nutrients and properties and its abilities to clean the body. When toasted, buckwheat is called Kasha. In Russia, Kasha is served with onions and brown gravy.

To Cook: There is a sweet spot for where your buckwheat will be tender enough to eat, but not mushy. Bring 2 cups of water to a boil in a medium saucepan with some salt. Stir in 1 cup of buckwheat and bring back to a boil. Keep the lid off. Once the buckwheat starts to expand and all the visible water is absorbed, turn down the heat to low and place the lid on the pot. Leave the buckwheat to cook for another 5 to 15 minutes, depending on the consistency you desire. Check it regularly. Buckwheat can be used in a tart, crepe, muffins, pancakes, waffles, salad, bread, and soup

Quinoa

Also low on the Glycemic Index, Quinoa originated in South America and has been a staple in the South American diet for centuries. More than a grain it is a seed relative of spinach, kale and Swiss chard. As a super food, it is low in calories and rich in dietary fiber and protein and low in calories.

Quinoa is also low on the glycemic index, as low as vegetables. And due to its fiber content, quinoa makes you feel full much faster. Its dietary fiber binds to fat and cholesterol, which causes your body to absorb less fat and cholesterol. The fiber found in quinoa also reduces the plaque build-up along your arterial walls, which reduces your risk of heart disease and stroke. Quinoa contains high quality protein and has a protein profile similar to cow's milk. It is an excellent source of iron, calcium, magnesium, B Vitamins and riboflavin.

(Be sure to rinse it several times before cooking to remove the bitter coating.)

To Cook: Rinse it well. There is a bitter coating on the tiny seed that needs to be rinsed away. When rinsing it, use a fine-mesh strainer. Combine 1 cup of quinoa with 2 cups of water in a medium saucepan. Bring to a boil. Cover, reduce heat to low and simmer until quinoa is tender, about 15 minutes. When cooked, drain the quinoa for 15 minutes; otherwise your dish will be watery. Return quinoa to the hot pot. This allows it to dry out. Quinoa tastes fabulous in salad, pudding, stuffing, sushi, cereal, cookies, pilaf, and risotto.

Teff

Teff has been a staple in the Ethiopian diet for thousands of years. It is an ancient North African cereal grass and a super food! The germ and bran, where the nutrients are concentrated, account for a larger volume of the seed compared to the more popular grains. It is also the world's smallest grain and is 40% resistant starch, meaning that half the calories consumed cannot be absorbed.

Resistant starch foods like teff can help you lose weight if you use it as a substitute for pasta. It's also low on the Glycemic

Index. What's unique about Teff is that it is packed with Vitamin C. Grains are normally devoid of this vitamin. Teff possess the eight essential amino acids a body needs in order to properly grow. Teff also helps manage the body's blood sugar levels and triggers bowel movements to perform properly.

It has a mild, nutty flavor and can be used to make polenta, cookies, breads, stews and so much more.

To Cook: Rinse teff under cold water. Add 1 cup of rinsed teff and 3 cups of water to a pot. Bring to a boil. Turn the heat to simmer, cover the pot and let cook for about 10 to 15 minutes. Turn off the heat, and let the teff sit for about 10 minutes. This allows the teff to absorb all the water. It should be sticky and nutty. Teff can be incorporated into muffins, scones, pie, pancakes, cake and even shortbread!

Wild Rice

Not far from our home is a Canadian aboriginal reserve called Curve Lake Reserve. Here wild rice is manufactured in small quantities and sold at our local farmer's market. This rice is absolutely delicious. You can smell the toasted grains while it's boiling in the pot.

Wild rice isn't really rice at all. It is the seed of a grass that grows in fresh water. It has twice the protein and fiber of brown rice, thus giving it a lower GI index. It is rich in antioxidants, possessing 30 times more than white rice, thus reducing the risk of cardiovascular disease. Due to its high fiber, wild rice also lowers bad cholesterol. It's good source of vitamins and minerals include Vitamins A, C and E, phosphorus, zinc and folate.

To cook wild rice, bring 3 cups of water to a boil and add 1 cup of rice. Reduce the heat and simmer on low for 40 to 45 minutes or just until kernels puff open. Uncover and fluff the rice with a fork. Drain off any excess liquid. This rice has a natural affinity to mushrooms. It can be served as a side dish or in soup, salad, pilaf, stuffing, casserole and pancakes.

Brown Rice

Because of its high fiber content, brown rice fills the stomach more quickly. This generally leads to automatic smaller meal portions, thus helping you inadvertently eat less. Brown rice is considered moderate on the Glycemic Index.

While requiring a long cooking time, brown rice is considered one of the world's healthiest foods. It is the whole grain with its inedible outer hull removed, while still retaining its nutrient-rich bran and germ. (White rice is both milled and polished, removing the bran and germ along with all the other layer-rich nutrients).

Some of the most popular varieties include: Long grain brown rice, with springy character, is well suited for casseroles and baked dishes. Medium grain brown rice is stickier and ideal for Spanish dishes like paellas. Short grain brown rice has creamy texture and can be used in risotto. Brown basmati rice is firm and has a dry consistency, ideal for biryanis and pilafs. Aromatic jasmine rice is moist and tender and good for Asian dishes and Kalijira rice grains are fast cooking and can substitute couscous-based dishes

One cup of brown rice provides your body with 80% of its daily manganese requirement. Manganese is important to help your body synthesize fats. Brown rice comes in short, medium and long lengths and in a whole bunch of different varieties with flavors and aromas. It is a good source of selenium, phosphorus, copper, magnesium, and niacin and fiber, fatty acids, amino acids and more. Due to its massive nutritional value, brown rice supports the prevention of ailments, including heart disease, cancers, diabetes, gallstones, decreasing asthma and the inflammation of rheumatoid arthritis.

To Cook: Rinse rice until the water runs clear. In a medium saucepan add 2 tablespoons of olive oil. Heat the oil, then add 1 cup of rice. This helps to build the flavor of the rice. Add 2.5 cups of water and a pinch of salt and bring to a boil. Reduce the heat to simmer, cover the pot and let simmer until the rice is tender, about 40 minutes. When the rice has finished cooking and the water has boiled off, let it rest with the lid on, for about 5 minutes. Brown rice can be utilized in sushi, risotto, as a side dish, in a pilaf or casserole, soup, salad, as a base in ingredient with a stir-fry or with Thai or East Indian curry.

Millet

Originating in China and making its way to Europe by 5000 BC, millet is a small-seeded grass, a cereal crop. Today it is revered in both India and in parts of Africa. Unfortunately, in North America it is primarily grown for birdseed.

Millet is highly underestimated and under-used in the kitchen. Considered an alkaline food with a moderate Glycemic Index, it is easily digested and has lots of fiber and low simple sugars. Some of its vitamins and minerals include Vitamin B3, copper, manganese, phosphorus and magnesium. This grain is high in fiber and so helps prevent gallstones and breast cancer.

Like all other grains, rinse millet under cold water before cooking to get rid of any dirt or debris. Add one-part millet to 2 parts water. Bring the water to a boil and reduce the heat to simmer. Cook millet for about 25 minutes or until the grain is fluffy like rice. It can be served as porridge, in bread, muffins, as a side dish, and in croquettes.

Corn

Yes, corn is a mysterious one, in deed. It is a dry fruit, popularly known as a grain and eaten as a vegetable. It is used in a plethora of gluten-free breads, pasta and prepared foods and so it is included. All varieties of corn – white, yellow, blue, purple and red – possess antioxidants. It's loaded with antioxidant phytonutrients, such as anthocyanins, beta-carotene, caffeic acid, coumaric acid, ferulic acid, lutein, syringic acid, vanillic acid, protocatechuic acid and zeaxanthin. The variety of corn determines its content and levels of antioxidants. While only small studied have been performed on corn with respect to its antioxidant power, research shows that this dry fruit often used as a grain is important in the reduction of risk for

Corn is also high in fiber, thus helping to reduce the risk of colon cancer and intestinal issues and high in B-complex vitamins (B1, B5 and folic acid).

When eaten in moderation, corn has also proved to be beneficial in blood sugar control in both type 1 and type 2 diabetes.

Amaranth

Considered a weed by much of the world, Amaranth was used by the Aztecs as a food staple. It is not really a grain, but rather a seed belonging to the Amaranthaceae family. This seed has a significant amount of the essential vitamins A, C, E, K, B5, B6, folate, niacin and riboflavin. These act as antioxidants, thus increasing energy and controlling hormones. It is also rich in lysine (an amino acid) calcium, potassium, iron, copper, magnesium, phosphorus and manganese, protein, dietary fiber, and amino acids — all essential for a healthy body. Lysine in particular is believed to help reduce the risk of cancer and lower bad cholesterol. Amaranth is also great in boosting the immune system. It helps fight off certain diseases such as cardiovascular disease and hypertension.

Amaranth's moderately high content of oxalic acid inhibits much of the absorption of calcium and zinc. It should be avoided or eaten in moderation by those inflicted with gout, kidney disorders or rheumatoid arthritis.

While packed with vitamins and minerals, Amaranth is high on the Glycemic Index, so eat in moderation and in small portions.

To Cook: 1 cup of amaranth to 3 cups of water. Bring to a boil, and then simmer for 25 minutes. The final consistency will be thick, like porridge. If you want to combine amaranth with another grain, substitute it with about ¼ of the other grain, then cook as you would for that grain. Amaranth can be added to risotto, salad, bread, or combined with other grains as a side dish.

Sorghum

Originating in Africa about 8000 years ago, Sorghum is a cereal grain used in Gluten-Free cooking. Because it doesn't possess an inedible hull like other grains, Sorghum is commonly eaten with all its outer layers, thereby providing your body with its nutrients. It is also grown from traditional hybrid seeds and so does not contain traits gained through biotechnology. It is non-transgenic (non-GMO). It is great for weight loss as Sorghum digests more slowly with a lower glycemic index, and so sticks with you a bit longer than other flours or flour substitutes. It also helps to speed up the metabolism and at the same time supports it. Sorghum contains a lot of magnesium and copper, minerals playing an important role in proper food metabolization. Packed with antioxidants, this cereal helps to reduce the risk of cancer development and cardiovascular disease.

Sorghum can be substituted for wheat flour in a variety of recipes. It's neutral, sometimes sweet and is easily adaptable. It improves the texture of recipes. This grain is also high on the Glycemic Index so consume in moderation and in small portions.

To Cook: Rinse, drain and pick through sorghum. Combine 3 cups of water or stock with 1 cup of Sorghum in a pot with a lid. Bring to a boil. Cover, reduce the heat to low and let simmer for about 50 to 60 minutes. Drain any excess water. Sorghum can be added to bread, salad, cookies, a pilaf and casserole, muffins, cake, cupcakes, and tabbouleh.

Chapter 8: Sugar Swaps: Low Glycemic Sugar Substitutes

One of the secrets to the Gluten-Free lifestyle for weight loss is to utilize healthy sugar substitutes in place of refined sugar and to refrain from artificial sweeteners. Look for "natural "sweeteners instead, ones that possess a low glycemic index.

Stevia: Glycemic Index 0

Stevia is a "sweet" sugar substitute. In fact, it is 300 times sweeter than sugar! It has been a staple in the South American diet for centuries. With zero calories and a glycemic index of zero, stevia has become a popular substitute for diets. Unfortunately, it possesses a slightly bitter after taste and so doesn't always feed one's sugar fix!

When baking, don't substitute stevia for sugar of the same measurement. It's best to only use stevia in baking recipes that have been designed for this substitute.

Buy only quality stevia. It comes in powder, syrup or liquid form.

Yacon: Glycemic Index 1

Extracted from the Yacon plant (a tuber), this South American sweetener has half the calories of sugar and a high concentration of indigestible inulin fiber, which means it breaks down slowly in the body. It's also high in potassium, calcium, phosphorous, iron and 20 amino acids! And above all, this sweetener is considered a prebiotic that heals the digestive system.

Agave Syrup: Glycemic Index 15

The Aztecs loved agave syrup, considering it a gift from the Gods that derives from the Blue Agave cactus plant. This is the same syrup that is fermented to produce tequila. Similar to honey in flavor, agave is half as sweet as sugar. This Aztec sweetener is rich in vitamins E, C, and D, calcium, iron, zinc and magnesium.

When baking use ¾ cup of agave syrup to every 1 cup of white sugar.

Comes in syrup form.

Lucuma: Glycemic Index 25

This substitute is made from the Peruvian lucuma fruit. One tablespoon of sugar has about 48 calories. Lucuma has 60! BUT...you tend to use half as much because of its intense sweet taste! It's a great substitute in recipes calling for brown sugar. Lucuma is also high in iron, zinc, potassium, calcium, magnesium, vitamin B3, beta carotene, and fiber.

Brown Rice Sugar: Glycemic Index 25

This sweetener's name says it all. It is made from boiled rice and has a thick, gooey consistency. Some of its many health benefits include B5, vitamin K, niacin, and thiamin.

Honey: Glycemic Index 30

Honey can help you lose weight. Since honey is sweet, you would think, at first, that it is an ingredient that causes weight gain, like refined sugar. But this is not the case. Honey actually has more calories than sugar. Honey possesses about 22 calories per teaspoon. The difference is that honey is a lot sweeter than sugar. As a result, people consume about half as much. So it becomes a better caloric tradeoff. This sweetener is also less processed. The refining process strips out the vitamins, minerals, proteins, and fiber once found in the sugar cane. Hence sugar becomes empty calories.

Honey is also processed, but naturally, by bees, leaving all the nutrients. Raw honey does not cause blood sugar spikes thus keeping insulin levels stable. It is anti-bacterial, anti-fungal and anti-viral. So the next time you have a cold, sip lemon-ginger tea with fresh lemon juice and fresh ginger, and use raw honey. Honey is also alkalizing for the body and aids in acid-indigestion. Research also shows raw honey reduces muscle cramps and cures insomnia. Vitamins B1, B2, B3, B5, B6, as well as vitamin C are found in honey, along with magnesium, potassium, calcium, sodium chlorine, copper, iron, manganese, zinc and phosphate. It's super healthy!

The biggest secret about raw honey? It helps to dissolve fat. In the morning consume 1 to 2 tsp. of raw honey in warm water with fresh lemon.

It is important to buy and use raw versus pasteurized honey. The pasteurization (heat treatment) process strips the honey of most of its health benefits.

Coconut Palm Sugar: Glycemic Index 35

Coconut palm sugar comes from the sap of the coconut tree. It has the same amount of calories as refined sugar but a lower glycemic index. This sweetener is also rich in magnesium, potassium, zinc and B vitamins.

Maple Syrup – Glycemic Index 58

My most favorite sugar substitute of all is Canadian maple syrup! It has become an integral aspect of my country's heritage and tourism, our "Canadiana". I have taken it for granted.

But it's probably one of the world's prized gems for the Gluten-Free weight loss and/or diabetic lifestyle plan.

According to an article on Diabetes Health, "Researchers from the University of Rhode Island have discovered that the syrup (produced in the northeastern United States and Canada) contains numerous compounds with real health benefits. In our laboratory research, we found that several of these compounds possess anti-oxidant and anti-inflammatory properties, which have been shown to fight cancer, diabetes and bacterial illnesses," said Navindra Seeram, an assistant professor of pharmacognosy (the study of medicines derived from natural sources) at the university and the study's lead author. Substances called polyphenols contained in the syrup might help control blood sugar levels, Seeram said. But that's not all. More than 50 beneficial compounds were found in maple syrup by researchers. Five of those compounds hadn't even been seen in nature before."

In a Toronto Star article dated March 12, 2013, Navindra Seeram explained that "the newly-discovered compounds found in maple syrup are types of lignans, also found in flax seed and whole wheat, a stilbene." Stilbene (or stilbenoids) is a secondary product of heartwood formation in trees, and in this case, maple trees. It acts like an antioxidant, similar to the antioxidants of the same chemical class as resveratrol and flavonoids found in grapes for wine. Silbeniods are considered as having anti-inflammatory, anti-cancer preventatives and antioxidant properties. Like wine.

So is maple syrup as healthy and as good for us as red wine? Some scientists believe that tapping causes the blood of the tree to secrete phenolics as a defense mechanism when wounded.

I was recently reintroduced to maple syrup and have discovered that it can add amazing complexity and dimension to Gluten-Free hors d'oeuvres, dressings, soups, entrees and, of course, Gluten-Free desserts. Just a few of the many classic partnerships include maple and bacon, maple and chipotle, maple and sage, maple carrot, maple apple, maple cranberry and maple syrup and lemon.

Maple syrup and wine have many commonalities. Like wine, small production maple syrup can express its somewhereness (referred to in France as 'terroir'). Each sugar bush (maple tree farm) is affected by its unique and identifiable geography, climate and soil conditions. The conditions create the distinctive character, intensity and flavor of the tree's blood, its sap. Weather conditions alter from year to year and so too does the sap's character and concentration. When syrup derives from the sap of the same maple trees in a sugar bush year after year for generation after generation, this is referred to as its "somewhereness." It is artisanal. One-of-a-kind. Unique. The sugar bush makes the syrup. The producer simply presents Mother Nature's gift to you. As consumers we are interested in the product's identifiable character yet yearly inconsistency.

Maple syrup's flavor and color not only vary from year to year, but also throughout each individual season. As the season progresses, its fructose and glucose levels rise; its sucrose levels slightly fall. The levels of other compounds like the minerals in the maple water also change throughout the season. At the beginning of the season, the syrup is often clear and slightly sweet. Later the syrup becomes darker and more caramelized.

Like wine, maple syrup can also be organic or not. In Canada strict government health and safety codes regulate this industry.

Large-scale production is the opposite of somewhereness. The sap from several sugar bush is gathered and boiled together. The aim is to produce a product of consistent color and flavor that creates a brand. In supermarkets these products are often marketed as artisanal, but are highly commercial and can contain preservatives.

Just as I advocate for beef, buy your maple syrup right from the farmers.

Like all products, pure maple syrup has a shelf life of about 1 year. Freezing can help to preserve its life and can later be used for cooking. Once opened, the container should be stored in the refrigerator.

Maple Syrup's color is not an indication of quality or purity. Color gives the consumer an idea of the syrup's intensity of flavor. Generally speaking, and each producer varies, the darker the color, the stronger the flavor. The intensity is expressed through grades.

Despite its sweetness, maple syrup is now considered the new super food, according to many new scientific studies.

Salad of Mixed Greens with Apples and Walnuts Drizzled in a Maple Syrup Dressing

Maple Dressing

¼-cup fat free or low fat mayonnaise

¼-cup pure Canadian maple syrup

3 tablespoons rice vinegar

½-cup vegetable oil

Salad

1 bag mixed greens

2 Granny Smith apples, peeled, cored, sliced

½-cup dried cranberries

½-cup chopped toasted walnuts*

*Toast walnuts in dry fry pan

In a bowl whisk all dressing ingredients until well blended.

Vegan Maple-Chipotle Roasted Butternut Bisque, Serves 4

1 1/2 large butternut squash

Olive oil as needed

Sea salt as needed

1-cup plain soymilk

1 chipotle pepper in adobo sauce

¼-cup maple syrup

½-cup of vegan sour cream

¼-cup vegan butter

Sea salt and butter to taste

Peel and cube butternut squash. Preheat oven to 375 F. Put cubes in a bowl and drizzle with olive oil. Toss around. Sprinkle with sea salt. Place the cubes on a lined baking sheet and roast until tender, about 45 minutes. Let cool. In a food blender add cubes with 1 cup plain soy milk (extra if you want a thinner soup). Add chipotle pepper in adobo sauce, pure maple syrup, vegan sour cream, softened vegan butter, salt and pepper to taste. Puree until smooth. Transfer mixture to a pot and heat.

When hot transfer to bowls. Garnish with a dollop of vegan sour cream and fresh herbs.

Suggested Wine: Pair this bisque with a semi sweet Riesling. This dish requires the wine's sweetness to cut through the heat and spice and to also harmonize with the natural sweetness in butternut squash and maple syrup.

Date Sugar: Glycemic Index 68

Made from dehydrated ground dates, this date sugar is packed with nutritional benefits, such as potassium, calcium, iron, magnesium, phosphorus, zinc, iron, copper, manganese and selenium.

Chapter 9: Get the Skinny on Fats

Over 15 years ago I became aware of Dr. Udo Erasmus, M.D. and his booked entitled 'Fats that Heal Fats that Kill'. This is a fantastic book that discusses research on common and lesser known oils with therapeutic potential, such as flax, hemp, olive, fish, evening primrose, borage, black currant and even snake oil! In his book, Dr. Erasmus also exposes the manufacturing processes that turns healing fats into killing fats. He explains the effects of these damaged fats on our bodies.

In your quest to lose weight through a Gluten-Free lifestyle, it's important to be aware of the fats that can heal your body and those that can kill.

We need fats to live and they are an important part of any healthy diet, including a Gluten-Free one. Fats provide essential fatty acids, which keep our skin soft, deliver fat-soluble vitamins and are a source of fuel to give us energy.

The problem is that we eat too much fat and too much bad fat. It's pretty simple. If you eat a diet high in fat (whether it's Gluten-Free or not) you are going to gain weight. The reason is that fat is calorie dense. Fat has 9 calories per gram where carbohydrates and protein have only 4 calories per gram. Alcohol has 7 calories per gram. Our obsession with fat adds more than visceral fat to our waistline. It triggers diseases and puts us at risk of heart disease, a plethora of cancers and type 2 diabetes.

Here's the secret, what is important to know. Good fats and bad fats all share the same amount of calories. So, it's important to also keep all fat consumption in moderation when aiming to lose weight. We only require about 10% of our calories to come from fat. Just be sure to eat healthy fats.

Fats deemed by some as 'bad' consist of saturated and trans fats. Saturated fats are believed to raise cholesterol levels. Trans fats are believed to also increase bad cholesterol and decrease good cholesterol. Saturated fats are found in butter, fatty meats, cheese and whole milk. Trans fats are found in processed foods.

If your recipes call for ingredients with saturated fat, choose healthier versions like raw and/or organic. Choose organic pork or beef, for example. If your recipe calls for butter, use butter. Just head to the health food store and choose raw, organic butter. While butter is a type of saturated fat, it's also loaded with nutrition. Butter is rich in Vitamin A, lauric acid, lecithin, anti-oxidants, Vitamins E and K, selenium, linoleic acid, Vitamin D, to name a few. Simply said, butter treats fungal infections, is essential for cholesterol metabolism, protects against free radical damage, fights cancer, builds muscles, boosts one's immunity and protects against tooth decay. Shall I go on? So why give up butter? Just choose healthy versions of this saturated fat and eat it in moderation or just on your fat-loading day of the week.

Unsaturated fats are healthy and support the heart, lower LDL (bad) cholesterol and raise HDL (good) cholesterol. Healthy fats come from monounsaturated and polyunsaturated varieties.

Polyunsaturated fats are those found in oily fish like sardines, anchovies, trout and salmon. Plant oils are also polyunsaturated. They include safflower seed and almond butter.

Monounsaturated fats are found in olive oil, some nuts (hazelnuts, macadamia nuts, almonds, pecans) and avocados. Research reveals that polyunsaturated fats (and to a lesser extent, monounsaturated fats) have shown to lower bad cholesterol levels, helping to keep your heart healthy.

Coconut oil is a funny one. While it has saturated fat, a type of MCT, it can also be dubbed as the new super food. Scientific research shows that lauric acid (in coconut oil's saturated fat) increases good HDL cholesterol. Coconut oil increases digestion and boosts thyroid function, metabolism, energy and endurance, among its many benefits.

Most exciting is a new clinical trial that was performed by the USF Health Byrd Alzheimer's Institute showing that coconut oil is now believed to be highly beneficial in treating Alzheimer's and, perhaps, other dementia. Again, choose organic, cold pressed versions.

Chapter 10: March to the Starch

Another secret to weight loss within the Gluten-Free lifestyle? Resistant starch! It is getting more attention of late as it has received praise from the Food and Agricultural Organization (FAO) and World Health Organization (WHO). In fact there have been hundreds of studies revealing that resistant starch is a healthy food group for weight loss and management, glycemic control and digestive health.

Simply put, resistant starch is a type of starch that moves completely through the small intestine without being digested. As a result these starches act like soluble fiber. They help to lower fat levels because they have less energy and consequently fewer calories than other starches. They assist the fermentation of good bacteria that can affect our hormones, body fat, and glucose and glycemic index levels in a way that encourages weight loss.

Research has shown that resistant starch foods have health benefits, such as:

- promoting satiation to encourage weight loss

- decreasing hunger to encourage weight loss

- affecting glycemic index levels to encourage weight loss

- positively affecting our hormones

- improving insulin resistance

- lowering insulin and glucose levels after meals

- making more butyrate than other prebiotics

- lowering the risk of bowel cancer

- bolstering immune system

- improving gastrointestinal health

- improving kidney health

Resistant starch takes a considerably longer time to digest. That means expanding as it soaks up fluids in your body stimulating satiety and giving you effective control over your appetite.

Here is a list of resistant starch foods to include in your Gluten-Free menu whenever possible:

Green Bananas (1 medium peeled, 4.7 g of resistant starch)

In North America we seem to only like to ripe bananas. But green bananas are an integral part of other cultural menus, such as in the Caribbean and Jamaica. Bananas contain inulin, a resistant starch that serves as a strong probiotic in the body, improving health gut flora as well as controlling blood sugar. I like to incorporate green bananas into bread. It's fabulous in shakes and frozen yogurt.

White Beans (1/2-cup, prepared, 4.5 g)

White beans offer a double benefit for the Gluten-Free eater. They are high in resistant starch. They also are low in fat. Beans reduce blood sugar, and create the fatty acid butyrate, which burns fat faster. Studies have shown that butyrate improves mitochondrial function in your cells, leading to a decrease in fat. If you are concerned about gas, fret not. The more beans you eat, the more your body will build up the good bacteria to digest them. I love to puree white beans with garlic, fresh lemon juice, Parmigiano-Reggiano and salt and pepper to taste. Spread the mixture on Gluten-Free toast. It is a tasty hors d'oeuvre. It can also be served as a dip with rice crackers.

Lentils (1/2-cup, 3.7 g)

Lentils are legumes, the seeds of plants whose botanical name is lens esculenta. In North America we consume green or brown lentils. But they are also available in black, yellow, red and orange. Lentils readily absorb the flavors of the other ingredients in a dish and they have high nutritional value, as well as being a high resistant starch with no fat! Lentils are a good source of cholesterol lowering fiber and prevent the blood-sugar level from rising after a meal. While giving the body energy, lentils also can help reduce the risk of coronary heart disease and cardiovascular disease. They are a good source of folate, copper, phosphorus, manganese, iron, protein, B1, zinc, potassium and vitamin B6. Before cooking lentils spread them out and remove any stones. Then wash them thoroughly. Place them in boiling water for 20 to 30 minutes, depending on their end use. Often this legume gets overlooked or type-casted in the roll as a soup and stew ingredient. But lentils can be used in making burgers, omelets, dips, chili, sloppy Joes, vegetarian Moussaka, tacos, Indian Mango Dal, risotto, salads and even cabbage rolls.

Yams (1/2-cup, cooked, 2.5 g)

I probably eat more sweet potato than yams. But yams are a resistant starch and certainly more enticing from this perspective. Yams are different than sweet potatoes. The flesh inside a sweet potato is orange. The flesh inside a yam is white to purple. Yam is the starchier and drier distant cousin of sweet potato. It originated in Africa where 95 percent of the crops are still grown. The rough scaly skin ranges from off-white to dark brown. Yams are low in fat and are a good source of vitamin C, B6, thiamin, manganese, copper and potassium. It is a healthy complex carbohydrate that helps the digestive tract and aids in decreasing the risk of obesity, heart disease and several forms of cancer.

We tend to stick to one yam dish – candied yams. But yams can be incorporated into the bean burrito, stews and soups, kebabs, Gluten-Free breads, mashed with potatoes, garlic and Parmesan and more.

Chickpeas (1/2-cup, prepared, 2.0 g)

I think my husband and I survive on chickpea dip called hummus with Gluten-Free tortilla chips. It certainly wards off hunger pains until dinner. In a food processor or blender combine 2 cups of canned chickpeas (drained and rinsed) with 3 tablespoons of tahini, 2 cloves of garlic, 2 tablespoons of lemon juice, ¼ cup of coconut or olive oil, and kosher salt and black pepper to taste. This Middle Eastern legume can also be used in salads, burgers, and soups. Chickpeas can also be pureed with yogurt and cumin and served as a dip. Besides being a resistant starch, chickpeas boost your energy, stabilize blood sugar levels and are high in protein and have a low glycemic index. They reduce bad cholesterol, aiding in the reduction of the risk of heart disease.

Green peas (1/2-cup, prepared, 2.0 g)

Green peas are not as powerful a resistant starch as green bananas, but they are packed with other nutrition that's hard to beat.

Green peas, in the legume family, are a nutritionally loaded addition to soups, salads, as a side dish, or in stir-fries and noodle dishes, to name but a few. They contain important fat-soluble nutrients like beta-carotene, vitamin E, omega-6 fatty acid and linoleic acid. Some other green pea health benefits include anti-aging, a strong immune system and high energy. These benefits come from their flavonoids (catechin and epicatechin), carotenoid (alpha and beta-carotene), phenolic acids (ferulic and caffeic acids) and polyphenols (coumestrol).

Due to their strong anti-inflammatory properties, vitamins C and E and Omega-3 fat, green peas help to prevent wrinkles, Alzheimer's, arthritis, bronchitis, and candida. They are high in fiber and so regulate the blood sugar level, aid in the reversal of insulin resistance (type 2 diabetes) and improve bowel health. With an abundance of vitamin B1 and folate, B2, B3, and B6, vitamin K (anchors calcium), green peas aid in the prevention of heart disease and osteoporosis as well.

When purchasing fresh green peas look for pods that are firm and smooth. They should have a medium green color and are flat. If the color is dark, yellow, whitish or specked with gray, avoid them.

Brown Rice (½ cup, cooked, 1.6 g)

Brown Rice is covered in Chapter 7.

Kidney Beans (1/2-cup, prepared, 1.4 g)

I've been studying the many benefits of beans, specifically kidney beans. When combined with rice, this legume provides an excellent source of protein – without the high calories and fat of red meat! In fact, one cup of kidney beans provides 15.3 grams of protein, 30% of one's daily requirement.

Like most beans, kidneys are also an excellent source of cholesterol lowering fiber. Hypoglycemic and diabetic friendly, these beans help to stabilize blood sugar levels after meals.

One of the best benefits of kidneys is that they are high in 'molybdenum.' Molybdenum is a trace mineral and an important part of the enzyme sulfite oxidase, which is responsible for detoxifying sulfites in the body.

One cup of cooked kidney beans supplies about 177.0% of our molybdenum daily requirement. I checked my multivitamin. It contains 8 mcg of this trace mineral. For the human being, 75 mcg of molybdenum is a daily requirement. So, kidney beans are now a part of my weekly Gluten-Free food repertoire.

Molybdenum is believed to help to protect the stomach and esophagus against cancers, aids in the absorption of iron and so helps to prevent anemia, as well as tooth decay. Molybdenum also aids in the metabolizing of fats and carbohydrates. (Other than kidney beans, other foods high in molybdenum are meats, buckwheat, barley, wheat germ, lima beans, sunflower seeds and dark green leafy vegetables.)

Most importantly, kidney beans are high in soluble and insoluble fiber. Soluble fiber produces a gel-like substance that increases stool bulk and therefore helps to prevent constipation.

When buying kidney beans at bulk food stores, look closely to ensure they are not cracked, thus indicating too much moisture content.

To prepare dried kidneys quickly and for culinary greatness, rinse the beans under cool water. Place them in a pot on a burner with just enough water to cover. Bring the water to a boil and then let the beans simmer for 2 minutes. Remove the pan from the heat. Let the beans stand in their liquid for two hours.

Remove the beans from this liquid. Discard the liquid. Rinse the beans under cool water again. Put them into a clean pot. Add 3 cups of water to every 1 cup of beans. Bring the water to a boil. Reduce the heat to simmer. Let the kidneys cook for another 1.5 to 2 hours until soft and done.

Quinoa (1/2-cup, cooked, 1.0 g)

Quinoa is covered in Chapter 7.

Potato (1/2-cup, cooked/mashed 0.6 to 0.8 g)

Despite the bad press, potatoes are a resistant starch packed with nutrients. Potato is rich in immune-boosting vitamin C and B, potassium, magnesium and iron. It contains a blood pressure lowering chemical called kukoamines, which the Chinese use in making teas for lowering blood pressure. And with 60 different kinds of phytochemicals and vitamins, the potato reduces the risk of cardiovascular disease and bad LDL-cholesterol and helps to keep arteries clear.

Did you know that one potato serves as 12 percent of your daily-recommended dose of fiber? They improve bowel health and support healthy digestion. Rich in vitamin B6, this tuber helps to reduce stress. Stress reduction aids in weight loss, as you already know.

Chapter 11: The Need for Speed

We know that weight loss is closely associated with our metabolism. What exactly is the metabolism?

Metabolism is the amount of energy or calories our body needs to maintain throughout the day. Everyone's metabolism is different and is affected by their body composition. People with greater muscle mass will have a higher metabolism. Those with less muscle have a slower one.

Those with greater muscle mass can consume more calories without gaining weight. Probably one of the most effective ways to speed up the metabolism is to exercise regularly incorporating both aerobic and anaerobic exercise, such as weight lifting.

The good news is that there are a few tips and ingredients and foods that you can incorporate into your Gluten-Free lifestyle to speed up your metabolism.

Secret 1: Exercise moderately and regularly:

Throughout my teens, 20's and 30's I was obsessed with staying thin, depriving myself of food, binge eating and working out like a maniac. When I hit my 40's and remarried and found happiness, I went in the opposite direction. I gave up exercise, ate and drank whatever I enjoyed and gained an enormous amount of weight. Now in my 50's I've finally found moderation. I have found a few girlfriends who also enjoy walking. This is so I am not tied to the schedule of just one person. I walk but 3 miles on each outing, and do this consistently. It is the consistency of my moderate walking that has contributed toward the shedding of my extra weight. On good days my girlfriend and I will walk faster, not longer.

Secret 2: Drink Less Alcohol:

As a food and wine writer, it's important that I recipe test and assess wines for my column. In the past I enjoyed a glass of wine with my meals -- sometimes 2 glasses. But I no longer drink wine every day. I assess wines, that is smell and taste them and then spittoon – spit them out. I now "drink" wine on occasion. Regular alcohol consumption sabotages weight loss. Alcohol stimulates the appetite causing us to eat more food during the meal. It also adds calories and slows the metabolism.

Secret 3: Sleep at least 7 to 8 hours per night:

The timing, duration, and quality of our sleep directly affects endocrine, metabolic, and neurohormonal functions related to our health. Proper sleep is vital in the control and management of our weight. Getting proper sleep decreases the risk of metabolic disorders such as insulin resistance and diabetes, to name but two.

Research also now reveals a link between our metabolism and sleep. Not getting enough sleep can slow one's metabolism. The quality of our sleep also orchestrates a symphony of hormonal activity tied to our appetite. Research on the hormones called leptin and ghrelin show that both can influence our appetite. And studies show that production of both may be influenced by how much or how little we sleep. Have you ever experienced a sleepless night and the next day your hunger never seems to be satisfied? This is a result of leptin and ghrelin at work.

Secret 4: Adding BCAA Powder to your shake.

BCAA stands for branched-chain amino acids. They can help repair and build muscle even when you can't make it to the gym! Muscle burns at least three times the number of calories as fat. This makes building muscle a priority for boosting the metabolism. BCAA supports our body repair and rebuilds muscle. Add 1000 mg of BCAA powder to your morning shake. Always consult your doctor before adding a new supplement to your diet, especially if you are taking medications.

Secret 5: Add cayenne pepper to your Gluten-Free dishes.

Cayenne contains capsaicin, a compound that stimulates the body's pain receptors, temporarily increasing blood circulation and metabolic rate. Studies have shown that eating hot peppers or cayenne can actually boost the metabolism for up to 3 hours and by up to 25%. Adding capsaicin to our diet is also healthy.

Capsaicin acts as a blood thinner, helping to prevent blood clots, which reduces the incidence of blood clotting related diseases. It is also an anti-inflammatory.

Secret 6: Eat Broccoli:

Broccoli is extraordinarily high in vitamins C, K and A. One serving of this green super food also provides the body with lots of folate and dietary fiber and antioxidants. Broccoli detoxifies the body, thus helping it function more efficiently and ultimately supporting weight loss.

Secret 7: Eat Apples and Pears:

State University of Rio de Janeiro research showed that women who ate three small apples or pears daily lost more weight than those who did not.

Secret 8: Eat calcium-rich foods:

Studies show that people who consumed about 1200 milligrams of calcium per day lost almost double the amount of weight than those who did not. Calcium-rich foods speed the metabolism. Calcium is also necessary for the grown and maintenance of our teeth and bones, nerve signaling, muscle contraction and the secretion of certain hormones and enzymes. Foods high in calcium include:

Calcium-rich foods to incorporate into your Gluten-Free lifestyle include:

- Dark leafy greens (kale, spinach, watercress, arugula, mustard greens)

- Low fat cheeses – partly skimmed mozzarella

- Low to no fat yogurt

- Chinese cabbage (bok choy)

- Okra

- Broccoli

- Green snap beans

- Almonds

- Canned sardines

- Flaxseeds

- Sesame seeds

- Rhubarb

- Fresh parsley, thyme, basil

- Garlic

Note: Be careful about taking calcium supplements. Too much calcium can lead to kidney stones, strokes and heart attacks. It's always best to attain vitamins and minerals through the foods we eat.

Secret 9: Eat foods high in Omega-3's:

Munching on foods high in omega-3 acids is the greatest way to speed up the metabolism. These acids reduce the production of a hormone called leptin, a chemical that slows the metabolism. Consume foods high in Omega-3 acids, such as nuts and seeds, hemp oil, flax seed oil, etc.

Secret 10: Consume Coconut oil:

From a medicinal standpoint, coconut oil is a super food. It is a rich source of good saturated fat with almost 90% of the fatty acids in it being saturated. The saturated fat contains Medium Chain Triglycerides (MCTs).

Every time you eat, the process of digesting food burns off at least 10 percent of the calories you consume. Try replacing fats with coconut oil and you will speed up your metabolism by 15%.That may not seem like much, but will make a difference over time. It has to do with coconut oil's molecular structure and how the body digests it. The medium chain triglycerides (MCTs) in coconut oil are shorter and more water soluble than in other oils like canola or olive oil.

The body processes coconut oil immediately and therefore there is less opportunity for the body to store it as fat. For this reason it boosts the metabolic rate.

Coconut oil can be used in shakes, salad dressings, as a butter substitute and in cooking and baking. Be sure to invest in organic cold pressed coconut oil.

I try to use this oil as a substitute for other oils in as many ways as I can. I add it to Indian and Thai-based curry, in homemade Gluten-Free banana bread, and vinaigrettes.

As an aside, I mix coconut oil with vitamin E and use it as a face and body moisturizer.

Secret 11: Eat avocadoes:

This creamy green fruit is high in the right fats, the monounsaturated ones, which help control the metabolic rate. It is also high in fiber, vitamins and minerals. On a daily basis and as a snack I enjoy a dip combining avocado with fat free Greek yogurt and eat it with raw vegetables.

Secret 12: Eat more soup:

Research shows that flavorful soup satisfies both our palate and stomach, providing a combination of liquid and solid foods. Soup (those without saturated fats) can speed up the metabolism and help the body burn fat.

Secret 13: Drink purified water:

A Germany study showed that drinking water speeds up the fat burning process. It also detoxifies the body, making it more efficient to burn fat and suppresses the appetite.

Secret 14: Have a cup of caffeinated coffee:

The caffeine in coffee speeds up the heart rate, which in turn boosts the metabolism for about 3 hours. An 8-ounce cup of coffee has about 100 milligrams of caffeine. You should not consume more than 300 milligrams of caffeine per day. And you should consult your doctor if you have any health or heart issues that could be affected by caffeine.

Keep in mind that dark coffees are not necessarily stronger in caffeine. The caffeine level is determined by the bean variety, bean roasting level and coffee making process.

Robusto coffee beans have double the amount of caffeine than Arabica.

Lighter roasted coffees have more caffeine than darker roasts. This is because the prolonged toasting or heating of the beans breaks down the caffeine molecules.

The grind and the brewing process also affect the level of caffeine in the coffee.

The longer the coffee is brewed, the higher the level of its caffeine. French pressed coffee has a higher caffeine level because it is left to sit for a longer period of time.

So espresso, while stronger tasting, has less caffeine than brewed coffee.

Secret 15: Drink tea:

I am addicted to tea, almost as much as I was to wine. In fact, in an effort to lose weight, I cut back tremendously on wine sipping and replaced the habit with sipping tea – all kinds of tea. I crave the tannin in black tea as it has helped to subside my craving for the tannin in red wine. It has helped tremendously.

True tea is made from the leaves of an Asian evergreen known as Camellia sinensis. White tea, green tea, oolong tea, and black tea all derive from this plant. They also contain caffeine and so speed up the metabolism. Many factors influence how much caffeine is present in plucked tea leaves, such as the growing region, plant variety, age, leaf-age, nutrients, rainfall and stress by pests. The final production of the leaves from plant to tea also affects the level of caffeine.

60

The entire tea preparing process also affects its caffeine level. The temperature of the water used, brewing time and whether the leaves are loose, bagged or strained, also play an important role in the tea's caffeine level.

Tea Variety and Caffeine Level per 8 Ounce Cup

- White tea; 30 to 55 mg

- Green tea; 35 to 70 mg

- Oolong tea; 50 to 75 mg

- Black tea; 60 to 90 mg

Secret 16: Drink Green Tea:

Green tea is often an ingredient in weight loss products because it has been proven to burn fat and calories and speed up the metabolism. It also proves endurance during exercise. Green tea contains epiogallocatechin 3-gallate, a powerful antioxidant that stimulates the metabolism and enhances fat burning.

Secret 17: Eat papaya

Papaya contains papain, an enzyme that improves protein digestion and absorption. This is key to boosting metabolism and burning fat. Try incorporating this exotic super food into your diet. It can be added to salads, baked goods, desserts, dressings, salsa and sauces.

Chapter 12: Craving Killer Secrets

Maintaining a lifestyle of any kind is relatively simple until the cravings for unhealthy foods arise. It's so difficult to think straight and refrain from indulging in foods that our body seems to desire (rather than need). We've all heard or read about the most common ways to curb cravings, such as banning foods from the house or shopping on a full stomach. Here are a few different secrets on how to curb the cravings:

Secret 1: The Pinching Effect

Acupuncturists believe that pressure points restore balance in your energy, as imbalances and blockages cause cravings. One acupressure technique is to pinch your nose or earlobes for 10 seconds. A study in the Journal of Alternative and Complementary Medicine showed that weight loss patients who used acupressure techniques were able to maintain their weight loss better than those who didn't.

Secret 2: Cut Out High Glycemic Foods in the Morning

High glycemic foods are rapidly digested and result in high fluctuations in blood sugar levels. They spike your insulin levels, which leave you with a drop later, causing you to crave more food. Refrain from using artificial sweeteners. On the other hand, foods with a low glycemic index produce a gradual rise in blood sugar and insulin levels and are therefore healthier.

Secret 3: The Trifecta Effect

Keeping your blood sugar stable throughout the day is the most important way to kill sugar cravings. Every 3 hours eat a mixture of Gluten-Free protein (like nuts) with low-glycemic carbohydrates and healthy fats. This trifecta will serve you all day by stabilizing your blood glucose.

Almonds are a healthy source of protein, low glycemic carbs and healthy fats.

Apples contain soluble fiber, which helps delay the absorption of sugar into the bloodstream. Eat the skin, as well. It provides a significant source of fiber.

Secret 4: Add Magnesium

Chocolate cravings can be a sign of a magnesium deficiency. So add more dark green vegetables like spinach to your diet. This will help kill your craving for dark chocolate. Keep in mind that dark chocolate consumed in moderation is also healthy.

Secret 5: Hide your yellow and orange plates

Research has shown that the colors red, yellow and orange, because they are found in nature, actually stimulate the appetite. So, hide these plates away and use blue plates instead. Blue is almost never found in nature and so helps to suppress the appetite.

Secret 6: Brush Your Teeth

When you're experiencing cravings, brush your teeth. You may also want to invest in mint flavored toothpaste. It helps to curb the cravings even more.

Secret 7: Control Your Salt

Salt fools our taste buds, raises blood pressure, and triggers our cravings for sodium-rich foods, like fast food and junk food. If you're craving salty snacks on a regular basis this may indicate that your body is releasing a hormone called gherlin. The hungrier you are the more gherlin your body releases. Caralluma fimbriata is a supplement that stops the production of gherlin and nips your salt cravings in the bud. Start with 50 mg twice per day.

Chapter 13: Be a Conscious Shopper

If you're recently new to the Gluten-Free diet, it can be confusing and frustrating in attempting to navigate labels. Many countries have Gluten-Free certification programs in place. If you hunt through the Gluten-Free section of your local health food store or supermarket, you'll spot the logo on products. Or ask an employee to help you identify the certification logo.

There are ingredients listed on labels that use scientific names for wheat, barley, or rye and so they contain gluten. So be watchful of these names.

Scientific terms for ingredients with gluten on a food label include the following:

Triticum
Triticum is a type of cultivated wheat species, generally known as the most common type of wheat called 'bread wheat.' So stay away from any labels using this word.

Triticum vulgare (wheat)

Triticale (cross between wheat and rye)

Triticum spelta (spelt a form of wheat)

Hordeum vulgare
Hordeum vulgare is the scientific name for barley.

Secale Cereale
Secale cereale is the scientific name for rye.

Forms of Wheat, Barley, Rye
There are ingredients and processed foods that are a form of wheat, barley or rye. They are as follows:

Semolina (made from wheat)

Bulgur (a form of wheat)

Malt (made from barley)

Couscous (made from wheat)

Farina (made from wheat)

Pasta (made from wheat unless otherwise indicated)

Seitan (made from wheat gluten and commonly used in vegetarian meals)

Wheat Starch

People with Celiac disease, wheat allergies or wheat intolerance should avoid any foods containing wheat starch. It is a powder manufactured by the removal of proteins, including gluten, from wheat flour. While most of the proteins and gluten are removed, some may still be present. People with Celiac Disease have reported their reaction to products containing wheat starch. This may be due to the fact that some mills may use the same machinery for processing starch and gluten. Wheat starch is used as a thickening agent and stabilizer in gravies and processed foods. Watch for the terms:

Wheat protein/hydrolyzed wheat protein

Wheat starch/hydrolyzed wheat starch

Wheat Flour

Watch out for ingredients and products containing:

Wheat flour/bread flour/bleached flour

Wheat or barley grass (will be cross contaminated)

Wheat germ oil or extract (will be cross contaminated)

Products and Ingredients that May Contain Gluten

Nowadays supermarket shelves are filled with ingredients that are produced around the world. So, it's best to check all labels to ensure your foods are free of gluten.

Some of the ingredients on this list may or may not include gluten. Be sure to check the manufacturer before consuming. Most manufacturers have websites on line.

Vegetable protein/hydrolyzed protein (can come from wheat, corn or soy)

Modified starch/modified food starch (can come from wheat)

Natural flavor (can come from barley)

Modified food starch

Hydrolyzed plant protein (HPP

Hydrolyzed vegetable protein (HVP)

Seasonings

Gravies

Vegetable starch

Dextrin and Maltodextrin (sometimes comes from wheat)

Flavorings

The terms 'natural flavor' or 'natural flavoring' refers to the essential oil or extract of any product through roasting, heating or enzymolysis. This can be the extract from spices, fruits, vegetables, edible yeast, herbs, bark, leaves and plants. So, be careful as the 'natural flavoring' in an ingredient or product may come from a grain with gluten. Flavorings can often come from wheat and rye. Smoky flavoring comes from the burning of woods, such as mesquite or hickory. But again, be careful. Barley malt flour may be used as a carrier ingredient to help capture the aromas and flavors of the smoke.

Alcohol-Based Extracts

Alcohol based extracts like vanilla are Gluten-Free. The reason is that the alcohol in these products is distilled. Pure distilled alcohol is free of gluten regardless of the starting ingredient. During distillation the liquid from a fermented grain mash is boiled and the resulting byproduct is vapor. The vapor is captured and cooled and becomes liquid again. Because protein doesn't vaporize there are no proteins in the cooled liquid or extract.

Caramel

Caramel comes from cornstarch and so is free of gluten. Watch out for European ingredients with caramel, however. In Europe the caramel can be derived from barley or wheat.

Frozen Fruits and Vegetables

Fresh fruits and vegetables are free of gluten, but watch out for frozen versions. Sometimes frozen fruits and vegetables can be packaged on the same equipment or lines as wheat products. Cross contamination can be an issue. The key is to buy fresh when possible. And read labels.

Fresh meat and fish are free of gluten. Often in supermarkets fresh fish, poultry and meat are already seasoned. Refrain from purchasing these products. Flour is often used as seasoning filler.

Dairy Products

Dairy products should be consumed in moderation. Not all milk and dairy-based products are free of gluten though. Plain milk and yogurt is Gluten-Free. But flavored versions may not be. Refrain from yogurts with granola and ice cream with cookie dough.

Cheeses are generally Gluten-Free unless they've been washed in a beer brine solution. Check with your cheese monger before purchasing.

Watch for Hidden Sources of Gluten

Here are a few main culprits:

Egg Dishes, Quiche, Scrambled, and Omelets: Be careful when ordering egg-based dishes while dining out. Chefs often add flour to eggs to give quiche, scrambled eggs and omelets firmness. Be sure to ask your server about the ingredients used in the restaurant's egg-based dishes.

Sauces, Soups, Gravies and Casseroles: Be careful when dining out and indulging in classic comfort foods that incorporate 'roux.' Roux is a smooth mixture of flour and fat like bacon fat or butter. It is often used as a thickening agent in the creation of gravies, sauces and soups. Gluten can be hidden in mac and cheese, pasta with Alfredo sauce, and gravies in potpies, casseroles, gumbos, soups and stews.

Breadcrumbs in Ground Meat: When shopping, be sure to watch out for breadcrumbs used in ground meat products. Hamburger patties, meatloaf, meatballs and cabbage often contain breadcrumbs. (You can make your own gluten-free Panko breadcrumbs by placing about 3 cups of Rice Chex Cereal in a plastic bag and rolling a pin over them to make coarse or fine crumbs.)

Vitamins, dietary supplements and pharmaceutical drugs: Gluten can be hidden and used as filler in vitamins, supplements and drugs.

Chinese Food: Unfortunately, some of the tastiest sauces used in Chinese cuisine have gluten like soy, oyster and bean sauces. They contain wheat.

Conclusion:

I really want to thank you for reading this book. I sincerely hope my words have provided value for you and make a difference for you in your life. If you did receive value from this book, I would like to ask a favor of you. (Know that you also have the right to decline this request.)

Would you be kind enough to leave a review for my book on Amazon.com?

If so please click the link below to leave a review.

http://understandpublishing.com/visit/loveyourreview/

THE END

JOIN OUR FACEBOOK CLUB!

http://theglutenfreeclub.net/facebook